GASTROINTESTINAL HEALTH MADE DELICIOUS THE ACID WATCHER DEIT COOKBOOK WITH 75+ TASTY RECIPES

CHRISTINA BUDD

TABLE OF CONTENT

Tips and Tricks for Staying on Track with the Acid Watcher Diet

Embracing a Healthy and Delicious Approach to Gut Health

INTRODUCTION

Welcome to "Gastrointestinal Health Made Delicious: The Acid Watcher Diet Cookbook with 75+ Tasty Recipes"!

If you're someone who suffers from acid reflux, heartburn, or other gastrointestinal issues, you know just how frustrating and uncomfortable it can be. But what if we told you that you could manage your symptoms and improve your gut health simply by changing the way you eat?

That's where the Acid Watcher Diet comes in. the Acid Watcher Diet is a scientifically-backed approach to eating that focuses on reducing acid reflux symptoms and promoting a healthy digestive system. And now, with this cookbook, you can enjoy delicious and satisfying meals that are also designed to support your gut health.

Inside, you'll find over 75 mouthwatering recipes that are easy to make and packed with flavor. From breakfast dishes like Blueberry Quinoa Pancakes and Huevos Rancheros to main courses like Turkey Meatballs with Zucchini Noodles and Sweet and Sour Chicken, there's something for everyone. And with plenty of vegetarian and gluten-free options, you'll be able to find meals that work for your dietary needs.

But this cookbook isn't just about delicious recipes - it's also about helping you understand how the foods you eat impact your gut health. You'll learn about the science behind the Acid Watcher Diet and how it can help alleviate acid reflux symptoms and promote overall wellness. Plus, you'll find tips and tricks for making healthier choices when you're eating out or cooking on the go.

So what are you waiting for? Whether you're new to the Acid Watcher Diet or you're looking for fresh and tasty meal ideas, this cookbook has everything you need to support your gastrointestinal health and enjoy delicious meals at the same time. Let's get cooking!

CHAPTER 1

Introduction to the Acid Watcher Diet

Understanding Acid Reflux and Gut Health

The Acid Watcher Diet is a dietary approach that focuses on reducing acid reflux symptoms and promoting gut health. A leading expert in acid reflux and its impact on overall health.

Acid reflux occurs when the stomach acid flows back into

the esophagus, causing symptoms such as heartburn, chest pain, and difficulty swallowing. In addition to these uncomfortable symptoms, acid reflux can cause damage to the esophagus and contribute to more serious health problems if left untreated.

The Acid Watcher Diet is designed to reduce acid reflux symptoms by limiting or avoiding certain types of foods that trigger acid reflux. Specifically, the diet focuses on reducing the intake of acid-forming foods and increasing the intake of alkaline-forming foods. Acid-forming foods include items such as coffee, chocolate, spicy foods, and acidic fruits like citrus. Alkaline-forming foods include fruits, vegetables, whole grains, and lean proteins.

The Acid Watcher Diet also emphasizes the importance of how we eat, in addition to what we eat. This includes eating slowly, chewing thoroughly, and avoiding large meals before bedtime. By making these changes to the way we eat, we can reduce the amount of acid that is produced in the stomach and lower the risk of acid reflux.

The Acid Watcher Diet has been shown to be effective in reducing acid reflux symptoms and improving gut health. By following the diet, individuals can experience relief from symptoms like heartburn, indigestion, and chest pain. Additionally, the diet can help improve overall digestive health, reduce inflammation, and even improve the quality of sleep.

Overall, the Acid Watcher Diet is an effective dietary approach for managing acid reflux and promoting gut health. By understanding the principles behind the diet and making simple changes to the way we eat, individuals can experience relief from uncomfortable symptoms and improve their overall digestive wellness.

CHAPTER 2

Breakfast and Brunch

Starting Your Day with Delicious and Digestive-Friendly Dishes

Breakfast and brunch are important meals of the day that set the tone for how we feel and function. For those with acid reflux, it's essential to start the day with a meal that won't trigger symptoms. In this chapter, we explore delicious and digestive-friendly breakfast and brunch options that adhere to the principles of the Acid Watcher Diet.

The first meal of the day should be easy to digest and avoid foods that increase stomach acid production. For breakfast, low-acid fruits like bananas and melons make a great addition to oatmeal or yogurt. Oatmeal is a great choice because it's high in fiber and can be made with non-dairy milk. For those who prefer savory breakfast options, scrambled eggs with spinach and avocado are filling and nutrient-dense.

Brunch is a perfect opportunity to get creative with recipes that incorporate alkaline-forming ingredients. Shakshuka, a Middle Eastern dish made with eggs and a tomato-based sauce, is a flavorful and filling option that can be modified to include alkaline vegetables like kale and broccoli. Smoothie bowls made with alkaline fruits and vegetables like kale, pineapple, and ginger are also a great brunch option that is both delicious and easy to digest.

One of the biggest challenges of the Acid Watcher Diet is finding alternatives to popular breakfast and brunch staples like coffee and pastries. Luckily, there are several delicious and digestive-friendly options available. Chamomile tea is a great alternative to coffee that is soothing to the digestive system. Baked oatmeal cups made with almond milk and low-acid fruits are a tasty option for those who crave something sweet.

In summary, starting the day with a digestive-friendly breakfast or brunch is essential for those with acid reflux. By incorporating alkaline-forming ingredients like fruits and vegetables and avoiding acid-forming foods, individuals can reduce their risk of symptoms and improve their overall digestive health. With these delicious and satisfying breakfast and brunch options, adhering to the principles of the Acid Watcher Diet has never been easier.

CHAPTER 3

Soups, Salads, and Appetizers

Light and Flavorful Meals to Soothe Your Stomach

Soups, salads, and appetizers are a great way to incorporate healthy and delicious ingredients into your diet while also being easy on the stomach. In this chapter, we explore a variety of soups, salads, and appetizers that are both flavorful and soothing for those with acid reflux.

Soups are a great option for those with acid reflux as they are typically easy to digest and can be made with alkaline-forming ingredients. Vegetable-based soups like butternut squash or tomato soup are both delicious and nutrient-dense. For a heartier option, chicken and vegetable soup made with homemade bone broth can be a comforting meal that is also beneficial for gut health.

Salads can also be a great way to incorporate alkaline-forming ingredients into your diet. A simple salad with mixed greens, low-acid fruits like berries, and a vinaigrette made with apple cider vinegar is a flavorful and refreshing option. Adding grilled chicken or salmon can make the salad more filling and provide additional protein.

Appetizers can be a challenge for those with acid reflux, as many popular options like cheese and crackers or spicy dips can be triggering. However, there are several tasty and digestive-friendly options available. Roasted sweet potato rounds with avocado and salsa are a flavorful and nutrient-dense appetizer that is easy on the stomach. Hummus made with chickpeas, tahini, and garlic is also a great option that is high in protein and fiber.

One of the biggest benefits of incorporating soups, salads, and appetizers into your diet is that they can help you eat smaller portions at meals, which is beneficial for those with acid reflux. By starting the meal with a small bowl of soup or a side salad, individuals can feel full and satisfied without overeating.

In summary, soups, salads, and appetizers are an excellent way to incorporate alkaline-forming ingredients into your diet while also being easy on the stomach. By choosing options made with nutrient-dense ingredients like vegetables, fruits, and lean proteins, individuals can improve their overall digestive health while also enjoying delicious and satisfying meals.

CHAPTER 4

Meat and Poultry

Satisfying and Nutritious Entrees for Any Occasion

Meat and poultry are excellent sources of protein, iron, and other essential nutrients that are important for overall health. However, they can also be problematic for those with acid reflux due to their high fat content and potential to trigger symptoms. In this chapter, we explore a variety of meat and poultry dishes that are both satisfying and nutritious while also being gentle on the stomach.

One way to make meat and poultry more digestive-friendly is to choose lean cuts and cooking methods that reduce the fat content. Grilling, baking, or roasting are all great options that allow excess fat to drip away from the meat. Choosing lean cuts like chicken breast, turkey breast, or lean cuts of beef or pork can also help reduce the fat content.

Marinating meat and poultry before cooking can also help to tenderize the meat and add flavor without relying on high-fat ingredients like butter or cream. Acidic ingredients like lemon juice, vinegar, or yogurt can help break down the meat fibers and add a tangy flavor.

Some popular meat and poultry dishes that are digestive-friendly include grilled chicken or turkey breast, turkey meatballs made with lean ground turkey and almond flour, and beef stir-fry made with lean sirloin steak and a variety of colorful vegetables. These dishes are all high in protein and nutrient-dense, making them excellent choices for those looking to maintain a healthy diet while also managing acid reflux symptoms.

It's also important to pay attention to portion sizes when it comes to meat and poultry. While these dishes are nutritious and satisfying, eating large portions can put a strain on the digestive system and trigger symptoms. Aim to keep meat and poultry portions to around 3-4 ounces per meal, and incorporate plenty of vegetables and whole grains to create a balanced and digestive-friendly meal.

In summary, meat and poultry can be a nutritious and satisfying addition to any diet, but it's important to choose lean cuts, cooking methods, and portion sizes that are gentle on the stomach. Incorporating a variety of colorful vegetables and whole grains can also help create a balanced and digestive-friendly meal that supports overall health and wellbeing.

CHAPTER 5

Fish and Seafood

Heart-Healthy and Digestive-Friendly Options for Seafood Lovers

Fish and seafood are great sources of protein and omega-3 fatty acids, which are essential for overall health. They are also easy to digest and make for great meals that won't upset your stomach. In this chapter, we'll explore some delicious and digestive-friendly recipes for fish and seafood that are perfect for any occasion.

- Lemon and Herb Salmon: This delicious recipe combines fresh lemon and herbs with omega-3 rich salmon for a light and flavorful dish that is easy on the stomach. Serve with a side of roasted vegetables or a quinoa salad for a complete meal.
- Shrimp and Quinoa Bowl: Quinoa is a great

source of fiber and protein, making it an ideal base for a healthy and filling meal. This recipe combines quinoa with sautéed shrimp, avocado, and cherry tomatoes for a nutritious and delicious bowl that is easy on the gut.

- Grilled Halibut with Mango Salsa: Halibut is a great source of lean protein and omega-3 fatty acids, making it a heart-healthy choice for any meal. This recipe pairs grilled halibut with a sweet and tangy mango salsa for a delicious and easy-to-digest dish.

- Tuna and Avocado Poke Bowl: This popular Hawaiian dish is a great option for seafood lovers who want something fresh and healthy. This recipe combines cubed tuna with avocado, cucumber, and brown rice for a nutrient-packed and satisfying bowl.

- Coconut Curry Shrimp: Curry is a great way to add flavor to any dish, and this recipe uses coconut milk for a creamy and delicious sauce. Paired with shrimp and vegetables, this dish is a great way to get in your daily servings of veggies while also enjoying a flavorful and digestive-friendly meal.

By incorporating these fish and seafood recipes into your meal planning, you can enjoy the health benefits of these nutritious foods while also supporting your digestive health.

CHAPTER 6

Vegetarian and Vegan

Plant-Based Dishes Packed with Protein and Flavor

For those who follow a vegetarian or vegan diet, it can sometimes be challenging to find meals that are both satisfying and nutrient-dense. This chapter offers a variety of delicious and filling plant-based options that are high in protein and bursting with flavor.

- Black Bean and Quinoa Bowl: This bowl is a perfect meal option for lunch or dinner. It's loaded with black beans, quinoa, sweet potatoes, and avocado, providing a balanced mix of carbohydrates, protein, and healthy fats.
- Chickpea and Spinach Curry: This creamy and flavorful curry is made with chickpeas, spinach, coconut milk, and spices. It's a great

option for a cozy dinner and can be served with rice or naan bread.

- Lentil and Vegetable Soup: This hearty soup is packed with lentils, vegetables, and spices. It's a perfect meal for a chilly day and can be easily made in a large batch for meal prep.
- Tofu Stir Fry: This stir fry features tofu, broccoli, peppers, and other veggies. It's a quick and easy meal that can be served over rice or noodles for a filling and satisfying dinner.
- Roasted Vegetable and Hummus Wrap: This wrap is made with roasted vegetables, hummus, and a whole-wheat tortilla. It's a tasty option for lunch or a light dinner and can be easily customized with different veggies or spreads.
- Vegan Chili: This chili is packed with plant-based

protein from beans and quinoa. It's also loaded with veggies, spices, and a touch of sweetness from maple syrup. It's a great option for meal prep or a cozy night in.

- Quinoa and Vegetable Stuffed Peppers: These stuffed peppers are filled with quinoa, veggies, and cheese or a vegan alternative. They make a satisfying and flavorful meal for lunch or dinner.
- Sweet Potato and Black Bean Enchiladas: These enchiladas are made with sweet potato, black beans, and a tasty enchilada sauce. They're easy to make and can be served with a side of rice or a salad for a complete meal.
- Spinach and Mushroom Lasagna: This lasagna is made with a creamy spinach and mushroom filling and is layered with noodles and cheese

(or a vegan alternative). It's a perfect option for a special occasion or a cozy dinner at home.

- Chickpea and Vegetable Curry: This curry features chickpeas, sweet potatoes, and other veggies in a flavorful coconut curry sauce. It's a filling and satisfying meal that can be served with rice or naan bread.

These plant-based options are packed with nutrients, protein, and flavor, making them a perfect addition to any meal plan or dietary preference.

CHAPTER 7

Sides and Snacks

Sides and snacks are often overlooked when it comes to gut health, but they can actually play a significant role in supporting a healthy digestive system. In this chapter, you will discover a variety of delicious and nutritious side dishes and snacks that are easy to make and will keep your gut happy.

Roasted Sweet Potato Wedges

Sweet potatoes are a great source of fiber and vitamins A and C, making them an excellent choice for gut health. These roasted sweet potato wedges are crispy on the outside and tender on the inside, and they are seasoned with a blend of spices that will leave your taste buds satisfied.

Quinoa and Kale Salad

Quinoa is a high-fiber, protein-rich grain that is gentle on the digestive system. In this salad, it is paired with kale, another gut-healthy ingredient that is rich in vitamins and minerals. The salad is dressed with a simple vinaigrette that adds a tangy and refreshing flavor.

Grilled Asparagus

Asparagus is a prebiotic food that feeds the good bacteria in your gut, helping to keep your digestive system in balance. Grilling asparagus gives it a smoky flavor and a tender texture that pairs well with a variety of main dishes.

Homemade Hummus with Crudites

Hummus is a versatile dip that can be made with a variety of beans and spices. In this recipe, chickpeas are blended with tahini, lemon juice, and garlic to create a creamy and flavorful dip that is perfect for pairing with raw vegetables like carrots, cucumbers, and bell peppers.

Baked Sweet Potato Chips

These crispy baked sweet potato chips are a healthier alternative to traditional potato chips. Sweet potatoes are sliced thin and then baked until they are crispy and golden brown. They are seasoned with a blend of spices that adds a savory and slightly sweet flavor.

Garlic Roasted Broccoli

Broccoli is a cruciferous vegetable that is packed with fiber, vitamins, and minerals. Roasting it with garlic and olive oil gives it a delicious and savory flavor that is sure to please even picky eaters.

Greek Yogurt Dip with Fresh Herbs

Greek yogurt is a good source of probiotics, which can help to support a healthy gut microbiome. In this recipe, it is blended with fresh herbs like dill and parsley to create a tangy and flavorful dip that is perfect for dipping vegetables or spreading on toast.

Roasted Brussels Sprouts with Bacon

Brussels sprouts are another cruciferous vegetable that is rich in fiber and nutrients. Roasting them with bacon adds a smoky and savory flavor that is sure to please. This dish is easy to make and is a great side dish for any meal.

Almond Butter Energy Balls

These no-bake energy balls are the perfect snack for when you need a quick burst of energy. They are made with almond butter, oats, and honey, and are packed with protein and fiber to help keep you full and satisfied.

Cucumber and Tomato Salad

Cucumbers and tomatoes are both low in calories and high in fiber, making them a great choice for gut health. This salad is dressed with a simple vinaigrette and is perfect for serving alongside grilled chicken or fish.

Incorporating these tasty and nutritious side dishes and snacks into your meals can help to support a healthy gut microbiome and keep your digestive system functioning properly.

CHAPTER 8

Sauces and Dressings

Flavorful and Digestive-Friendly Condiments for Every Dish

Sauces and dressings can make or break a meal. Not only do they add flavor and depth to a dish, but they also have the ability to impact our digestive health. Many store-bought options are high in sugar, preservatives, and other additives that can trigger acid reflux and other digestive issues. The good news is that making your own sauces and dressings is simple, and allows you to control the ingredients and flavors.

In this chapter, you will learn how to make a variety of sauces and dressings that are both delicious and digestive-friendly. From classic vinaigrettes to creamy dips, these recipes will elevate any meal while also supporting gastrointestinal health.

Some of the recipes featured in this chapter include:

- Classic Vinaigrette: A simple yet flavorful dressing made with olive oil, vinegar, Dijon mustard, and herbs.
- Lemon Tahini Dressing: A creamy and tangy dressing made with tahini, lemon juice, and garlic.
- Roasted Red Pepper Sauce: A versatile sauce made with roasted red peppers, garlic, and olive oil that can be used as a dip, spread, or sauce.
- Cilantro-Lime Crema: A creamy and zesty dressing made with Greek yogurt, cilantro, lime juice, and garlic.
- Avocado-Lime Dressing: A rich and creamy dressing made with

avocado, lime juice, and honey.

- Balsamic Glaze: A sweet and tangy glaze made with balsamic vinegar and honey that is perfect for drizzling over roasted vegetables or grilled meats.

Each recipe is accompanied by detailed instructions and tips for customization. You will also learn about the specific digestive benefits of some of the ingredients used, such as ginger and turmeric.

By learning to make your own sauces and dressings, you can take control of your digestive health and elevate the flavor of your meals.

CHAPTER 9

Desserts

Desserts are often associated with being unhealthy and harmful to the digestive system. However, this does not have to be the case. In this chapter, you will find a selection of delicious and gut-healthy desserts that will satisfy your sweet tooth without causing digestive discomfort.

- Berry Chia Seed Pudding: This creamy and delicious pudding is packed with fiber, omega-3 fatty acids, and antioxidants from the chia seeds and berries. It is also free from dairy and gluten, making it a perfect dessert for those with dietary restrictions.

- Chocolate Avocado Mousse: This decadent dessert is made with avocado, which is high in healthy fats and fiber, and cocoa powder, which is rich in antioxidants. It is also free from refined sugar, making it a healthier alternative to traditional chocolate mousse.
- Almond Flour Brownies: These brownies are made with almond flour, which is gluten-free and high in protein and healthy fats. They are also sweetened with coconut sugar, a natural sweetener that is lower on the glycemic index than regular sugar.
- Grilled Pineapple with Coconut Whipped Cream: Grilling pineapple enhances its natural sweetness and adds a smoky flavor.

Served with coconut whipped cream, this dessert is a tropical treat that is rich in fiber and vitamin C.

- Apple Crisp: This classic dessert is made with oats, which are high in fiber, and apples, which are rich in antioxidants and fiber. It is sweetened with maple syrup, a natural sweetener that contains antioxidants and minerals.
- Banana Ice Cream: This creamy and delicious ice cream is made with frozen bananas, which are high in fiber, potassium, and vitamin C. It is a healthier alternative to traditional ice cream and can be topped with nuts or berries for added flavor and nutrition.
- Chocolate Covered Strawberries: Strawberries are low in calories and high in

antioxidants and vitamin C. When dipped in dark chocolate, they become a decadent dessert that is both delicious and nutritious.

- Lemon Poppy Seed Cake: This gluten-free and dairy-free cake is made with almond flour and coconut oil, which are high in healthy fats and fiber. It is sweetened with honey and flavored with lemon and poppy seeds, making it a refreshing and delicious dessert.
- Cinnamon Apple Chips: These crispy and sweet apple chips are a healthy and easy-to-make snack that can also be used as a dessert. They are made with cinnamon, which has anti-inflammatory properties, and are a good source of fiber and vitamin C.
- Chocolate Banana Bread: This gluten-free

and dairy-free banana bread is made with almond flour and sweetened with maple syrup. It is also packed with fiber, potassium, and healthy fats from the bananas and almond flour. The addition of cocoa powder makes it a rich and indulgent dessert.

These gut-healthy dessert options are not only delicious but also nutritious, making them a guilt-free treat that will not cause digestive discomfort. By incorporating these desserts into your diet, you can satisfy your sweet tooth while also promoting a healthy gut.

CHAPTER 10

Eating Out and On-the-Go

Tips and Tricks for Staying on Track with the Acid Watcher Diet

One of the biggest challenges of following any diet is staying on track when eating out or grabbing a quick meal on-the-go. This is especially true for those following the Acid Watcher Diet, as many common restaurant foods and fast food options can be high in acid and trigger acid reflux symptoms. However, with a little bit of planning and knowledge, it is possible to enjoy dining out and staying on track with the Acid Watcher Diet.

In this chapter, we will explore some tips and tricks for eating out and on-the-go while following the Acid Watcher Diet.

- Research restaurant menus beforehand: Before heading out to eat, take some time to research restaurant menus online. Look for items that are low in acid and avoid anything that is known to trigger your acid reflux symptoms. Many restaurants nowadays offer gluten-free and dairy-free options, so it's worth asking about these as well.

- Ask for modifications: Don't be afraid to ask your server for modifications to dishes. Ask for sauces and dressings on the side, substitute high-acid foods for lower-acid alternatives, and ask for grilled or steamed options instead of fried.
- Avoid trigger foods: While it's important to stay mindful of acid levels in foods, it's equally important to avoid trigger foods that are known to exacerbate acid reflux symptoms. Some common trigger foods to avoid include

spicy dishes, citrus fruits, tomatoes, and chocolate.

- Be mindful of portion sizes: Restaurant portions can often be larger than what we would typically eat at home, which can be problematic for those with acid reflux. Consider splitting an entree with a friend, or ask your server for a smaller portion.
- Pack snacks for on-the-go: When traveling or running errands, it's a good idea to pack some snacks that are Acid Watcher Diet-friendly. Some great options include sliced fruits and vegetables, nuts, and low-acid granola bars.
- Choose wisely at fast food chains: While fast food is generally not recommended for those following the Acid Watcher Diet, there are some options that can

work in a pinch. Look for grilled chicken sandwiches or salads with low-acid dressing options, and avoid fried foods and high-fat options.

By following these tips and tricks, it's possible to enjoy dining out and staying on track with the Acid Watcher Diet. Don't be afraid to ask for modifications and be mindful of trigger foods and portion sizes. With a little bit of planning, you can still enjoy delicious meals while supporting your gastrointestinal health.

CHAPTER 11

Conclusion

Embracing a Healthy and Delicious Approach to Gut Health

In this final chapter of the Acid Watcher Diet Cookbook, we will summarize the key principles of the diet and provide some practical advice for maintaining a healthy gut and overall wellness.

Throughout the cookbook, we have emphasized the importance of adopting a diet that is rich in whole, unprocessed foods and low in acidic and inflammatory ingredients. By following the Acid Watcher Diet, you can support your gastrointestinal health, alleviate acid reflux symptoms, and reduce the risk of chronic diseases.

In conclusion, we encourage you to embrace a healthy and delicious approach to gut health. The recipes in this cookbook are designed to be both satisfying and nourishing, and we hope that you have discovered some new and tasty ways to incorporate digestive-friendly ingredients into your meals.

However, we recognize that following a new diet can be challenging, especially when it comes to eating out or when you are on-the-go. That is why we have provided some tips and tricks in the previous chapter to help you stay on track with the Acid Watcher Diet, even when you are not in control of the ingredients.

Ultimately, the key to maintaining a healthy gut and overall wellness is to make mindful food choices, to listen to your body, and to prioritize self-care. We hope that this cookbook has inspired you to take a step towards optimal health and to continue exploring the many delicious and nutritious options that are available to you.

GLOSSARY

Glossary of Terms for Gastrointestinal Health Made Delicious: The Acid Watcher Diet Cookbook with 75+ Tasty Recipes

- Acid Reflux: A condition where the stomach acid flows back into the esophagus, causing heartburn, regurgitation, and discomfort.
- Antioxidants: Nutrients that prevent or reduce damage to cells caused by free radicals in the body.
- Esophagus: The muscular tube that connects the throat to the stomach.
- Gastroesophageal Reflux Disease (GERD): A chronic digestive disorder that occurs when stomach acid flows back into the esophagus, causing

inflammation and damage.

- Gut Microbiome: The collection of microorganisms that live in the digestive tract and play a crucial role in digestion, immune function, and overall health.
- Heartburn: A burning sensation in the chest that often occurs after eating or when lying down.
- Inflammation: A natural response of the body's immune system to injury or infection that causes redness, swelling, and pain.
- Laryngopharyngeal Reflux (LPR): A type of acid reflux that affects the throat and voice box, causing hoarseness, coughing, and other symptoms.
- pH: A measure of acidity or alkalinity of a solution, with a pH of 7 being neutral, below 7

being acidic, and above 7 being alkaline.

- Probiotics: Beneficial bacteria that live in the gut and promote digestive health.
- Reflux: The backward flow of stomach acid or food into the esophagus.
- Sphincter: A circular muscle that regulates the opening and closing of a tube or passage, such as the lower esophageal sphincter (LES) that controls the flow of stomach contents into the esophagus.
- Ulcer: A sore or lesion that develops in the lining of the stomach or small intestine, often caused by infection or long-term use of nonsteroidal anti-inflammatory drugs (NSAIDs).
- Vegan: A person who avoids all animal products, including meat, dairy, and eggs.

- Vegetarian: A person who does not eat meat but may consume dairy and eggs.